Mediterranea Cookbook

A Superlative Guide To Understanding The Concepts Of The Mediterranean Diet With Delicious Recipes And A Meal Plan For A Healthy Lifestyle

Sophie Hill

TABLE OF CONTENTS

INTRODUCTION

Thank you very much for purchasing this cookbook. Foods allowed on this diet include vegetables, nuts and fresh fruits, fish, poultry, whole grains, skim milk, yogurt, and olive oil. From time to time both eggs and red meat are recommended. Fresh raw food is the main attraction of this diet; its main methods of cooking on the grill and in the oven. Salads are also common dishes, and desserts should be based on mixed fruit. Natural seasonings are also important in this eating habit since garlic and onions are essential for flavoring naturally, as well as fresh herbs such as parsley, oregano and basil. I hope you enjoy recreating my recipes and that they can conquer your palate.

Enjoy your meal!

BREAKFAST RECIPES

.

Avocado ice cream

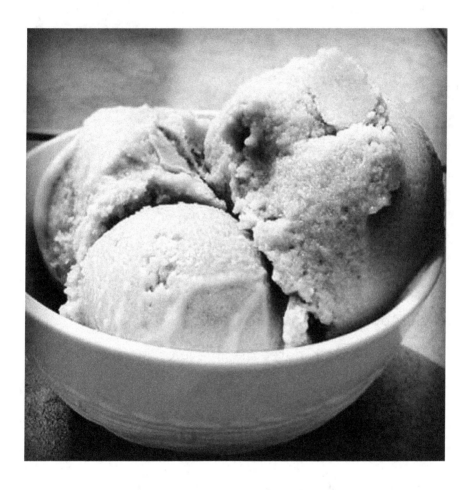

- cooking time 5mins
- serving 1
- calories 100

ingredients

- 1 avocado
- ½ lime
- 60 ml agave syrup
- 125 ml of coconut milk
- a pinch of salt

preparation

1. Halve the avocado, remove the stone, remove the pulp from the skin
2. Add agave syrup and puree
3. Occasionally puree the lime juice and coconut milk. Salt
4. Put the mixture in the ice cream maker or layer in a bowl
5. Put it in the freezer for 30-40 minutes

Banana blueberry porridge

- cooking time 10mins
- serving 1
- calories 597

ingredients

- 1 piece of banana (approx. 140 g)
- 60 g blueberries
- 50 g oat flakes (whole grain)
- 75 ml milk (low-fat 1.5% fat)
- 1 teaspoon honey
- 15 g almonds

preparation

1. Put the oat flakes, milk and 125 ml water in a saucepan and bring to the boil briefly over high heat.
2. Always stir well so that nothing burns.

15

3. Let everything soak briefly over low heat.

4. Put the porridge in a bowl and mix with honey.

5. Place the sliced banana and blueberries on the porridge and sprinkle with almonds if you like.

6. Mix and enjoy everything to eat.

Banana peanut shake

- cooking time 5mins
- serving 1
- calories 244

ingredients

- 1 piece of banana (approx. 140 g)
- 0.5 piece of apple (approx. 70 g)
- 1 tbsp peanut butter (natural)

preparation

1. Chop the fruit
2. Put the peanut butter and 100 ml water in a blender and mix well.

Banana French toast

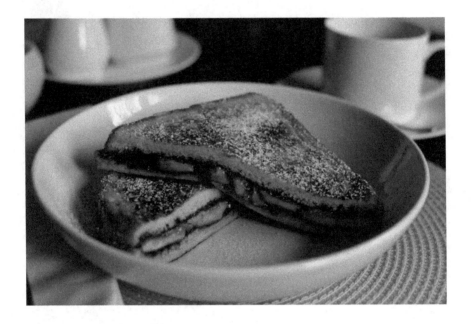

ingredients

- 2 slices of toast bread (whole grain)

- 1 piece of banana (approx. 140 g)

- 50 ml milk (low-fat 1.5% fat)

- 1 tbsp wheat flour (whole grain)

- 1 pinch of iodine salt

- 1 pinch of cinnamon

- 1 pinch of nutmeg

- 1/2 tbsp coconut oil

- 1/2 teaspoon honey

preparation

1. Finely mash the banana and mix well with the milk, flour, salt, cinnamon and some grated nutmeg.
2. Turn the slices of bread in it and let them steep briefly on each side (approx. 30 seconds).
3. Place a coated pan with a little coconut oil and fry the bread until golden brown on both sides.
4. Serve with fresh fruit, a little cinnamon and a little honey and enjoy.

LUNCH RECIPES

Cauliflower soup

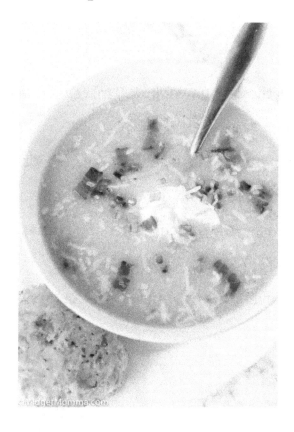

- cooking time 15mins

- servings 1

- calories 375

ingredients

- 1/2 cauliflower (approx. 390 g)

- 75 g sheep cheese

- 2 tsp vegetable broth

preparation

1. Cook the cauliflower in 400 ml vegetable stock until soft.
2. Puree half of the vegetables in a blender.
3. Then put it back in the broth and let it boil briefly.
4. Cut the sheep's cheese into small cubes and add to the soup.
5. Stir several times until the cheese has melted.

Broccoli on cheese

- cooking time 37 mins
- servings 1
- calories 579

ingredients

- ½ tbsp olive oil
- 50 g bacon (cubes)
- ½ piece of onion (30 g)
- green peppers (pickled) (approx. 20 g)
- pieces of garlic clove
- 100 g cream cheese
- ½ tbsp tomato paste
- 20 ml milk (low fat 1.5% fat)
- ½ piece of broccoli (approx. 180 g)
- 1 pinch of iodine salt
- 1 pinch of black pepper

preparation

1. Heat the oil in a pan, fry the bacon lightly, then add the onion, chopped peppers and finally the finely chopped garlic in this order.

2. Deglaze with milk.

3. Add the cream cheese and tomato paste and stir.

4. Pour in broccoli.

5. First thinly cut the stalk, then the florets with the stem down and season with salt and pepper.

6. Cook for 5 minutes with the lid on.

Bulgur salad with zucchini and carrot

- cooking time 20mins
- servings 1
- calories 277

ingredients

- 40 g bulgur
- ½ piece of zucchini
- 1 piece of carrot
- 1 tbsp apple cider vinegar
- 1 tbsp linseed oil
- 1 pinch of cumin
- ½ bunch of peppermint
- ½ bunch of parsley
- 1 pinch of iodine salt
- 1 pinch of pepper

preparation

1. Prepare bulgur according to the package instructions.
2. Wash the zucchini, halve and cut into thin slices.
3. Peel and wash the carrot and cut into fine sticks.
4. Wash parsley and peppermint, shake dry and chop.
5. For the vinaigrette, mix oil and apple cider vinegar and season with spices.
6. Add peppermint and parsley.
7. Fry the vegetables for about 4 minutes while turning and season with iodine salt and pepper.
8. Finally, fold the vegetables into the bulgur and serve with the vinaigrette.

Colorful bratwurst skewers

- cooking time 20mins
- servings 1
- calories 601

ingredients

- 150 g bratwurst
- 1 piece of apple
- 1 piece of onion (red)
- 1 tbsp rapeseed oil
- 1 tbsp sweet mustard
- 1 tbsp apple juice
- 1 pinch of black pepper
- ½ piece of zucchini

preparation

1. Wash, quarter and slice the apple.
2. Wash the zucchini, cut in half and also cut into slices.

3. Peel and cut the onion into eighths.

4. Halve the sausage crosswise and stick alternately with apple, courgette and onion pieces on skewers.

5. Whisk rapeseed oil, sweet mustard and apple juice and season with pepper.

6. Then brush the skewers with it and cook on the hot wire rack for 8-10 minutes, turning several times.

DINNER RECIPES

Vegetarian pasta Bolognese

- cooking time 20mins
- servings 1
- calories 600

ingredients

- 60 g of pasta
- ½ onion
- 100 g soy mince
- 1 tbsp flaxseed (crushed)
- 50 g of pureed tomatoes
- 20 g dried tomatoes
- 1 tbsp pine nuts
- 2 tbsp parmesan
- 1 tbsp coconut oil

preparation

1. Cook the pasta according to the instructions on the packet.

2. Heat coconut oil in a pan.

3. Chop the onions and fry them in the pan with soy mince and pine nuts.

4. Add the linseed, dried and pureed tomatoes and stir the sauce.

5. Mix the pasta and sauce and top with the parmesan.

Baked eggplant

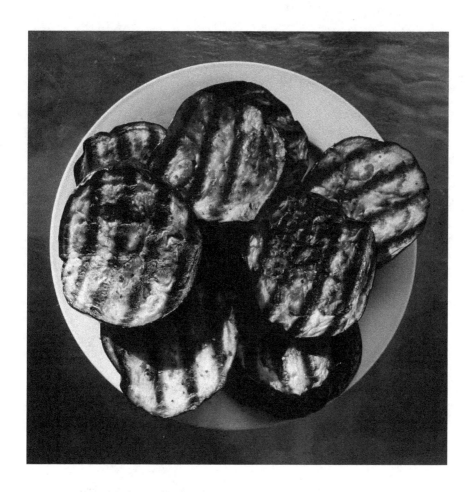

- cooking time 20mins
- servings 1
- calories 300

ingredients

- 1 large eggplant
- ½ paprika
- 4 cherry tomatoes
- 6 olives
- 1 tbsp olive oil
- 40 g feta
- salt and pepper

preparation

1. Cut the aubergine lengthways and remove the pulp.
2. Chop the pulp, peppers, tomatoes and olives into small pieces.
3. Mix the mix with the oil in a bowl, season with salt and pepper and then fill the eggplant halves.
4. Crumble the feta and crumble over the filled aubergine halves.
5. Place on a baking sheet and bake in the oven for 20 minutes at 200 ° C - then serve.

Tuna wrap

- cooking time 20mins
- servings 1
- calories 599

ingredients

- 1 piece of tortilla wrap (approx. 60 g)
- 1/2 piece of avocado (approx. 80 g)
- 50 g tuna (can)
- 30 g cream cheese
- 1/2 piece of onion (approx. 30 g)
- 30 g shrimp
- 1 tbsp chilli sauce

preparation

1. Cut the avocado into thin wedges.
2. Brush the wrap with cream cheese and top with tuna.

3. Cut the onion into thin rings, mix with the prawns and place on a wrap.

4. Drizzle with hot or sweet chilli sauce depending on your taste.

5. Fold the lower edge of the wrap inwards and fold the wrap together.

Curd dumplings with berries

- cooking time 20mins
- servings 1
- calories 599

ingredients

- 250 g curd cheese / low-fat quark
- 2 eggs
- 10 g psyllium husks
- 25 g of erythritol
- 30 g of wheat flour
- 150 g raspberries

preparation

1. Mix all ingredients with a hand mixer and let soak in the refrigerator for 10 minutes.
2. Bring water to a boil in a saucepan and then turn the temperature down - the water should no longer boil when the dumplings are added.

3. Shape the mixture into dumplings and fill with the berries.

4. Put the dumplings in the water and let it simmer for about 10 minutes.

5. Serve on a plate and garnish if you like.

Vegetarian stuffed mushrooms from the grill

- cooking time 20mins
- servings 1
- calories 193

ingredients

- 6 mushrooms (approx. 120 g)
- 100 g of cottage cheese
- 20 g cream cheese
- 1 clove of garlic
- 1 pinch of iodine salt
- 1 pinch of black pepper

preparation

1. Clean the mushrooms, carefully twist out the stems, cut off the ends and cut finely.
2. Mix the cottage cheese and cream cheese in a bowl, add the crushed mushroom stalks and season to taste.

3. Then peel the garlic, chop it finely and mix it with the cream.

4. Pour the cream into mushrooms and grill over low heat until lightly browned.

POULTRY, SALAD AND SMOOTHIE

Spicy carrot cocktail with nasturtiums

- Cooking time 15 to 30 min
- Servings 4

ingredients

- 20 g nasturtium (with flowers; or watercress; 0.5 bunch)
- 1 clementine
- 100 ml carrot juice (without sugar)

Preparation steps

1. Wash nasturtiums and shake dry well. Put 1-2 beautiful flowers aside, roughly chop the rest of the cress.
2. Halve the clementine and squeeze out. Mix the juice with the cress, carrot juice and ice cubes in a blender. Pour into a glass, pour in mineral water and garnish with capuchin flowers.

Strawberry tiramisu

- cooking time 5 mins
- servings 1
- calories 400

ingredients

- 500 g strawberries
- 250 g low-fat quark
- 250 g sour cream
- 50 g xylitol
- 150 g ladyfingers
- 1 lemon

preparation

1. Puree 200 g strawberries and set aside.
2. Cut the remaining strawberries into small cubes and mix with the xylitol, sour cream and low-fat quark.

3. Line a baking dish with ladyfingers and drizzle with lemon juice.

4. Apply a layer of the cream on top.

5. Then add a layer of strawberry puree.

6. Repeat steps 3 - 5.

Peanut butter smoothie

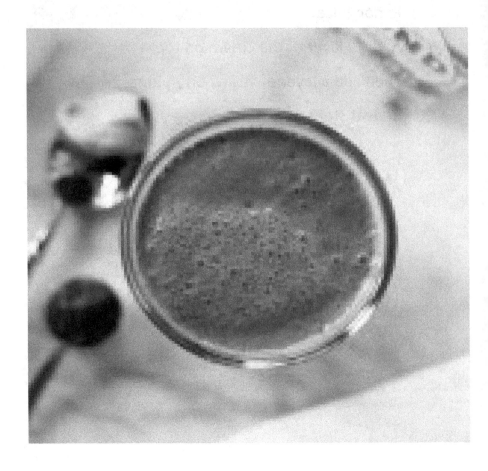

- cooking time 5 mins
- servings 1
- calories 223

ingredients

- 130 ml milk (low-fat 1.5% fat)
- 100 g plain yoghurt
- 1 tbsp peanut butter
- 50 ml of water

preparation

1. Put all the ingredients mentioned in a blender and blend until a creamy consistency has formed.

Frozen yoghurt with berries

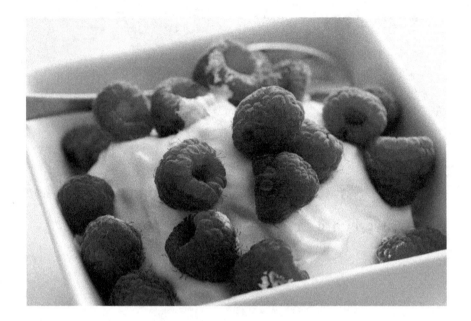

- cooking time 15 mins

- servings 1

- calories 120

ingredients

- 100 g natural yoghurt

- 200 g frozen berries

- 3 teaspoons of honey

preparation

1. Puree the natural yoghurt, berries and honey until a creamy mixture is obtained

2. Thanks to the frozen berries, the ice cream is ready to eat immediately

Fruity watermelon lemonade

- cooking time 5 mins
- servings 1
- calories 89

ingredients

- 125 g watermelon
- 200 ml of water
- 2 teaspoons of lime juice
- 1 teaspoon lemon fruit juice
- 1 teaspoon honey

preparation

1. Cut the watermelon into small pieces.
2. Puree the watermelon with lemon fruit juice, lime juice, water and honey in a blender. If the consistency is too firm, fill up with water.
3. Pour into a glass and enjoy.

Fruity salad with strawberries

- cooking time 20 mins
- servings 1
- calories 240

ingredients

- 100 g strawberries
- 25 ml of water
- 1 teaspoon balsamic vinegar
- 1 teaspoon olive oil
- 1 teaspoon honey
- 1 pinch of iodine salt
- 1 pinch of pepper
- 30 g rocket
- 25 g sheep cheese

preparation

1. Wash, clean and halve the strawberries.

2. Puree 25 g strawberries with water, balsamic vinegar, olive oil and honey and season to taste with salt and pepper.

3. Wash and clean the rocket.

4. Roughly dice the sheep's cheese and place in a bowl with the remaining strawberries and rocket.

5. Finally, drizzle the dressing over the salad.

Fruity watermelon salad

ingredients

- 250 g watermelon
- 150 g lamb's lettuce
- 50 g parmesan cheese
- 20 g pomegranate
- 4 walnuts
- 4 peppermint leaves
- ¼ bunch of parsley
- 1 teaspoon lemon fruit juice
- 1 teaspoon olive oil
- 1 pinch of iodine salt
- 1 pinch of pepper

preparation

1. Cut watermelon into small cubes.
2. Wash the lamb's lettuce and arrange on a plate.
3. Pour the watermelon, parmesan, pomegranate and walnuts over the salad.

4. Wash and chop the peppermint and parsley.

5. Mix lemon fruit juice with olive oil to a dressing, fold in the herbs and pour over the salad just before serving.

6. Season to taste with spices.

VEGETABLES RECIPES

Linguine with morels and asparagus

- cooking time 20mins
- servings 2
- calories 490

ingredients

- 320-400 g linguine (thin ribbon noodles)
- 100 g morels (fresh)
- 6 stick (s) asparagus (green)
- 100 ml veal jus (also available in delicatessen shops)
- 300 ml whipped cream
- 1 cl Madeira
- Parsley (chopped)
- butter
- Sea salt (from the mill)
- Pepper (from the mill)

preparation

1. Clean the morels, cut them in half and briefly wash them in water. Peel the asparagus at the lower ends, cut away the woody parts and cut the stalks into fine slices. Sweat the asparagus in a little butter, add the morels and deglaze with the Madeira. Pour veal jus and whipped cream on top and let everything boil down. Meanwhile, cook the linguine in salted water until al dente, drain and stir into the sauce. Season with sea salt and pepper and stir in the chopped parsley.

Zucchini Tagliatelle

ingredients

- 400 g zucchini
- 400 g tagliatelle
- 1 onion
- 2 toe (s) of garlic
- 1 pinch of nutmeg
- Herbs (fresh, as desired, e.g. basil, sage, etc.)
- 100 g parmesan (or sheep cheese)
- Olive oil (for the pan)
- salt
- pepper

preparation

1. Slice the zucchini into fine strips with a potato peeler. Peel the onion and the garlic cloves and chop them into fine cubes.
2. Cook the tagliatelle according to the instructions on the package.

3. Heat olive oil in a pan and sauté the onion and garlic until translucent. Add the zucchini strips. Season with salt, pepper and nutmeg.

4. Add the cooked tagliatelle, toss it through once, mix in the fresh herbs and season with grated Parmesan or diced sheep's cheese to taste.

Fried radicchio

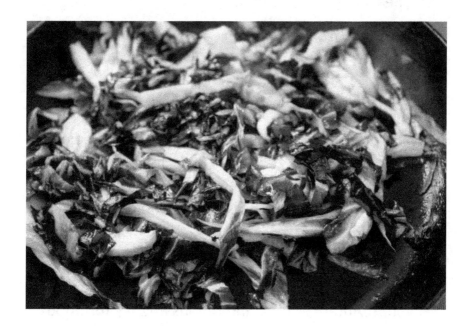

- cooking time 15mins

- servings 4

- calories 278

ingredients

- 750 g radicchio

- 4 onions

- 2 cloves of garlic

- 2 tbsp pine nuts

- 5 tbsp olive oil

- Sea salt (from the mill)

- Pepper (from the mill)

preparation

1. For the fried radicchio, first, clean the radicchio, remove the outer leaves and quarter lengthways. Cut out the stems. Eighth the onions and finely chop the garlic cloves.

2. Heat half of the oil in the pan and sweat the garlic in it. Add pine nuts and onions and fry for about 3 minutes, stirring constantly. Add the washed, well-drained radicchio and fry over low heat for about 5 minutes. Season the fried radicchio with salt, pepper and the remaining olive oil.

SEAFOOD RECIPES

Smoked trout spread

- cooking time 19mins
- serving 4
- calories 100

ingredients

- 1 cup of creme fraiche
- 3 eggs (hard-boiled)
- 2 trout (smoked)
- 3 tbsp herbs (chopped)
- pinch of pepper
- 1/2 cup of sour cream
- 1 squirt of lemon juice
- salt

preparation

1. For the smoked trout spread, peel the hard-boiled eggs cut them finely and place in a bowl. Chop the trout fillets and add.

2. Mix with creme fraiche and sour cream to make a spreadable fish spread. Finally, season with a splash of lemon juice and the chopped herbs.

3. Season to taste with salt and pepper and leave the smoked trout spread in the refrigerator for about 60 minutes.

Tuna salad with beans

- Preparation time 5mins
- Cooking time 15mins
- Servings 2

Ingredients

- 2 can (s) of tuna (Mexican)
- 1/2 bell pepper (yellow)
- some iceberg lettuce (cleaned and washed)
- tomato
- tbsp vinegar (preferably white wine vinegar)
- 1 tbsp olive oil
- 1 pinch of sugar
- salt
- Pepper (freshly ground)

preparation

1. For the tuna salad with beans, chop up the iceberg lettuce, mix with vinegar, salt, pepper, a pinch of sugar and oil. Arrange on plates, place the tuna in the centre, garnish the edge with thinly sliced paprika, quarter the tomatoes and place on top of the tuna. Sprinkle with pepper all around.

Pizza toast

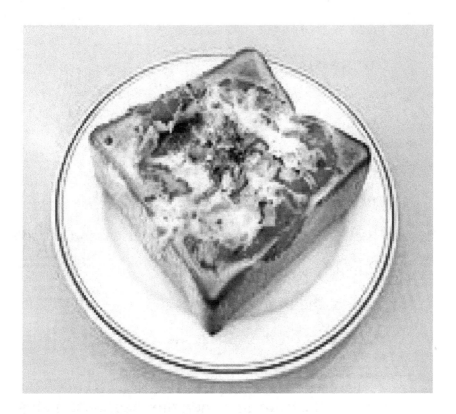

- cooking time 60mins

- serving 2

- calories 120

ingredients

- 1/4 stick (s) salami

- 1 pkg of pizza cheese

- 1 can (s) of tuna
- Pizza seasoning
- 1/2 can (s) of corn
- toast

preparation

1. Cut the salami into small pieces.
2. Then mix all the ingredients together and season with pizza seasoning.
3. Preheat the oven to approx. 200 ° C.
4. Place toast on the baking sheet and distribute the well-mixed ingredients on the bread.
5. Put it in the oven and when the cheese has melted and the bread are lightly browned, the pizza toasts can be enjoyed!

Breakfast with salmon trout and egg dish

- cooking time 20mins
- serving 4
- calories 300

ingredients

- 2 slices of rye bread (or wholemeal toast)
- 2 organic eggs (size M)
- 2 tbsp cream cheese (natural)
- 4 slice (s) of salmon trout (pickled)
- some butter
- salt
- Pepper (freshly ground)
- Sprouts (for garnish)

preparation

1. For breakfast with salmon trout and egg dish, toast the bread first. Lightly whisk the eggs and prepare

an egg dish in a little foamed butter, season with salt and pepper.

2. Brush the bread with cream cheese, spread the egg dish on top and cover with the pickled salmon trout. The breakfast of salmon trout and scrambled eggs with sprouts garnish.

MAIN AND SIDE DISH

Caprese

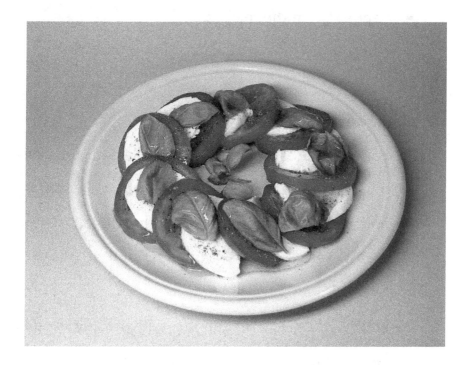

- cooking time 15 mins
- serving 4
- calories 675

ingredients

- 2 pieces of cheese (mozzarella)
- 4 tomato (s)
- Basil leaves

- Salt (from the mill)
- Pepper (from the mill)
- olive oil

preparation

1. For the Caprese, cut the mozzarella and tomatoes into slices. Then place a slice of mozzarella, tomato and basil leaves on top of each other directly on the plates. Season each with pepper and drizzle with olive oil.

2. Finally, sprinkle the Caprese with freshly ground sea salt and drizzle with a little olive oil.

Green beans and carrot soup

- cooking time 60 mins
- serving 5
- calories 222

ingredients

- 250 g green beans
- 3-4 carrots
- 1 pc onion
- 1 l vegetable soup (soup cubes)
- 30 g butter
- 3 tbsp flour
- parsley
- salt
- pepper

preparation

1. For the green beans and carrot soup the diced onion in the butter fry light, dust with the flour and pour in the vegetable soup.

2. Add the cleaned and sliced carrots. Clean the beans and cut them into thirds and add them to the soup.

3. Cook covered for about 45 minutes on a low flame.

4. The green beans and carrot soup with parsley refine and possibly season with salt and pepper.

Potato and rocket salad

- cooking time 15 mins
- serving 4

ingredients

- 800 g potatoes (greasy and cooked)
- 100 g rocket
- 1 teaspoon mustard
- 150 g onions (finely chopped)
- 100 ml of pumpkin seed oil
- 100 ml white wine vinegar
- 200 ml beef soup (warm)
- salt
- pepper
- sugar

preparation

1. For the potato and rocket salad, mix the mustard with the pumpkin seed oil, vinegar, warm beef

soup, salt, pepper and a little sugar. Slice the still-warm potatoes into leaves and add a little salt.

2. Cut the rocket and mix with the finely chopped onions in the marinade. Then mix with the potatoes.

Wild garlic spaetzle

- cooking time 15 mins
- serving 4

ingredients

- 400 g of flour
- 170 g wild garlic
- 4 eggs
- 300 ml of water
- salt
- Butter (to the pan)

preparation

1. Rinse the wild garlic leaves with cold water, shake dry and chop very finely.
2. Mix all ingredients into a dumpling dough and pour through a dumpling sieve into boiling salted water.
3. Let simmer for about 5 minutes, then strain.
4. Toss the spaetzle in a little butter.

Zucchini turrets

- cooking time 5 mins
- serving 4

ingredients

- 1 zucchini (small)
- 4 tomatoes (ripe)
- 2 pieces of mozzarella
- olive oil
- Seasoned Salt
- Basil (fresh)

preparation

1. For the courgette turrets, cut the courgette into 1 cm thick slices, season with salt and fry in olive oil in a pan.
2. Turn the slices over and top with a slice of tomato and mozzarella each. Cover the pan so the cheese melts.
3. Pepper and top with a fresh basil leaf.

DESSERT RECIPES

Pear with cream cheese

- Cooking time 30mins
- Servings 4

ingredients

- 2 pears
- 30 g cream cheese (leaner, with herbs)
- Lemon juice (some)
- 1 tbsp walnuts
- 1 tbsp pistachios

preparation

1. For the pear with cream cheese, peel and halve the pears, remove the core with a spoon and drizzle with a little lemon juice.
2. Mix the cream cheese with the herbs and spread it in the hollows of the pear.
3. Chop the walnuts and pistachios into small pieces. Then roll the pears outside in the nut pieces.

Ricotta cream

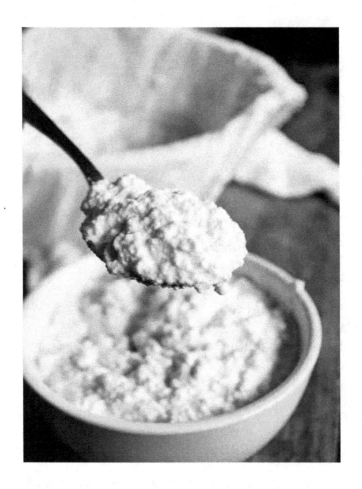

ingredients

- 250 g ricotta

- 250 g low-fat yoghurt

- 2 tbsp sugar (or as you like)

- 2 teaspoons Bourbon vanilla sugar (or as you like)
- Fresh fruits or cookies (for decoration)

preparation

1. For the ricotta cream, mix the ricotta with the yoghurt.
2. Then add sugar and vanilla sugar.
3. Mix everything again and serve the ricotta cream with fruit, biscuits, etc.

Yoghurt cream

ingredients

- 1/4 l milk
- 30 g corn starch
- 50 grams of sugar
- 1 pc egg
- 1/4 l cream
- various fruits (as desired)
- 1/4 l yoghurt

preparation

1. For the yoghurt cream, bring the milk to a boil. Mix the maizena with the yolk, sugar and some cold milk and add to the boiling milk. Then let it cool down. Stir in the yoghurt spoon by spoon and finally fold in the stiff cream.

2. Fill the yoghurt cream alternately with fruit puree in bowls and serve decorated with cream and fruit.

Chocolate cake

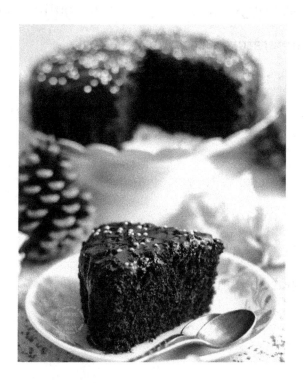

ingredients

- 200 g granulated sugar

- 200 g margarine (or butter)

- 200 g flour (smooth)

- 1 packet of baking powder

- 3 eggs

- 3 tsp cocoa powder

- 3 teaspoons of water

preparation

1. Beat eggs with sugar and butter at room temperature until frothy.

2. Sieve the baking powder into the flour (this way there are no lumps in the dough). Mix both with the egg mixture.

3. Mix cocoa with water and fold into the chocolate cake mixture.

4. Bake the chocolate cake at 160 ° C (hot air) for about 25 minutes.

SNACKS AND

APPETIZER

Vegetarian wraps

- cooking time 15 mins
- servings 4

ingredients

- 4 pieces of finished wraps
- 2 handfuls of lettuce
- 250 g of grated cheese
- 1 can (s) of beans
- 1 can (s) of corn
- 5 pcs. Tomatoes

preparation

1. Wash the beans, corn and lettuce for the vegetarian wraps.
2. Chop the tomatoes, puree a little and season well. Spread all ingredients, except for the salad, on the wraps and place in the preheated oven at approx. 150 ° for 10 minutes.
3. Finally, fill the vegetarian wraps with the salad and serve.

Paprika chips from the oven

- cooking time 15 mins
- servings 2

ingredients

- 2 potatoes (medium)
- 1 tbsp olive oil
- 1 teaspoon paprika powder
- salt .

preparation

1. For the paprika chips, peel the potatoes from the oven and cut into thin slices with the paring knife. Line a baking sheet with parchment paper. Brush the baking paper thinly with olive oil. Place the potato slices on top and brush lightly with olive oil.

2. Sprinkle with paprika powder and salt. The pepper chips baking in a preheated oven at 220 ° C, 6 minutes until golden brown.

Avocado dip

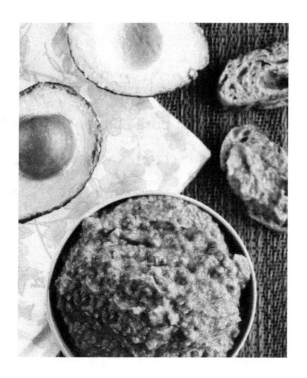

- cooking time 15 mins
- servings 2

ingredients

- 1 avocado (up to 2, ripe)
- 1 tbsp sour cream
- garlic

- salt

- pepper

preparation

1. For the avocado dip, peel the avocados and remove the stone . Mash or puree the pulp with a fork.
2. Stir in a little sour cream and season the avocado dip with freshly chopped garlic, salt and pepper.

Breaded zucchini

- cooking time 15 mins
- servings 2

ingredients

- 2 zucchini (unpeeled)
- 1 egg (whisked)
- 1 tbsp parsley (smooth, chopped)
- 2 tbsp breadcrumbs
- 2 tbsp olive oil
- 1 tbsp lemon (juice)
- salt
- Pepper (freshly ground)

preparation

1. Cut the zucchini into slices, season the zucchini slices with salt and pepper.
2. Mix the egg and parsley together. Dip the zucchini slices in it, then turn in breadcrumbs.
3. Fry until golden brown in hot oil. Drain on kitchen paper and drizzle with lemon juice.

CONCLUSION

Congratulations on making it to the end.

The Mediterranean diet offers a simple cuisine but rich in imagination, flavors, colors, scents and memories, enhancing all aspects of a healthy diet. It is an ethical option that preserves the traditions and customs of the peoples of the Mediterranean basin. The Mediterranean tradition offers a cuisine that supports the taste and spirit of those who live in harmony with nature.

Good luck!

CPSIA information can be obtained
at www.ICGtesting.com
Printed in the USA
BVHW091428300421
606211BV00006B/962